Simple Thoughts from a Chaotic Mind

A Collection of Stories and Essays from My Life with a Craniofacial Syndrome

Ellie Rose McCullagh

Booky-Books No. 1
RIT Press
Rochester, New York

Published and distributed by:
RIT Press
90 Lomb Memorial Drive
Rochester, New York 14623
https://press.rit.edu

Printed in the United States of America

ISBN 978-1-956313-29-1 (print)

We gather on the traditional territory of the Onöndowa'ga:' or "the people of the Great Hill." In English, they are known as Seneca people, "the keeper of the western door." They are one of the six nations that make up the sovereign Haudenosaunee Confederacy.

We honor the land on which RIT was built and recognize the unique relationship that the Indigenous stewards have with this land. That relationship is the core of their traditions, cultures, and histories. We recognize the history of genocide, colonization, and assimilation of Indigenous people that took place on this land. Mindful of these histories, we work towards understanding, acknowledging, and ultimately reconciliation.

Designed by Marnie Soom

Ellie,

By the time you turn eight, you will realize that you look different, and that different must be "bad." You dream of the day when you will one day be just as "normal" as everybody else, and you'll start to read books about people whose lives are very different from your own.

Before you turn ten, you will realize that people are mean and that, despite what people say, words can actually hurt you. That precious smile of yours will learn to hide behind walls, and those bright blue eyes—though they see much—will cost you any pride you have in your appearance.

When you're twelve, you'll start to have crushes and be reminded—yet again—that you're different. You'll spend hours comparing yourself to your peers, wondering why your friends are having first kisses while you're on the sidelines, concluding that it must be because of your face.

You couldn't be more wrong.

You are so beautiful. Your smile is contagious and your personality is so big and bright that it is what people notice first—not your face. You'll have gone through hell and back before you're sixteen years old, but somehow you'll make it. One day, you won't see the scarred cheeks or the crooked teeth in the mirror's reflection. You'll see the sum of many parts—and you'll call her pretty.

I know you distance yourself from the world because you don't want to get hurt again and when people ask questions, it is a sharp reminder that you will never be normal. You're still vulnerable to life's cruelties and it will be years before you take your guard down. I also know that with grace, time, and strength, you will become a force to be reckoned with.

You will do amazing things, Ellie Rose.

Sincerely,

A Friend

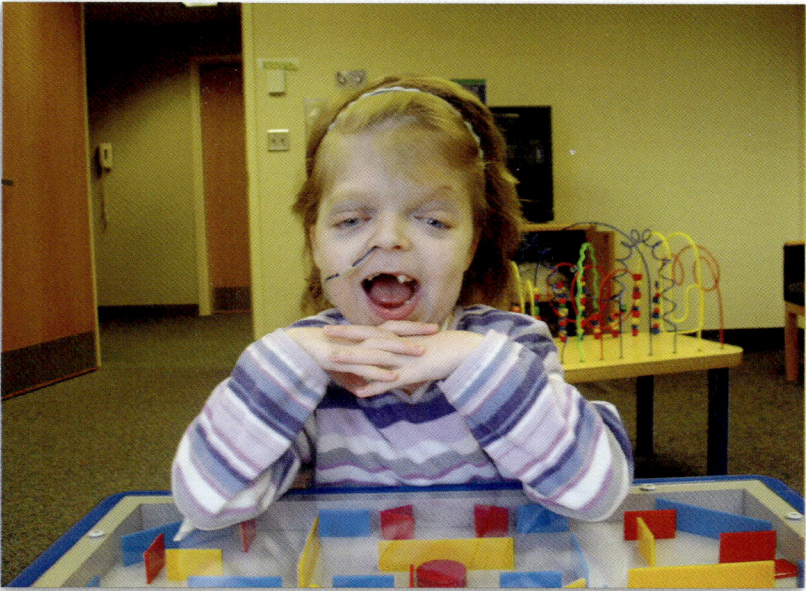

Ellie in a hospital waiting room (2004)

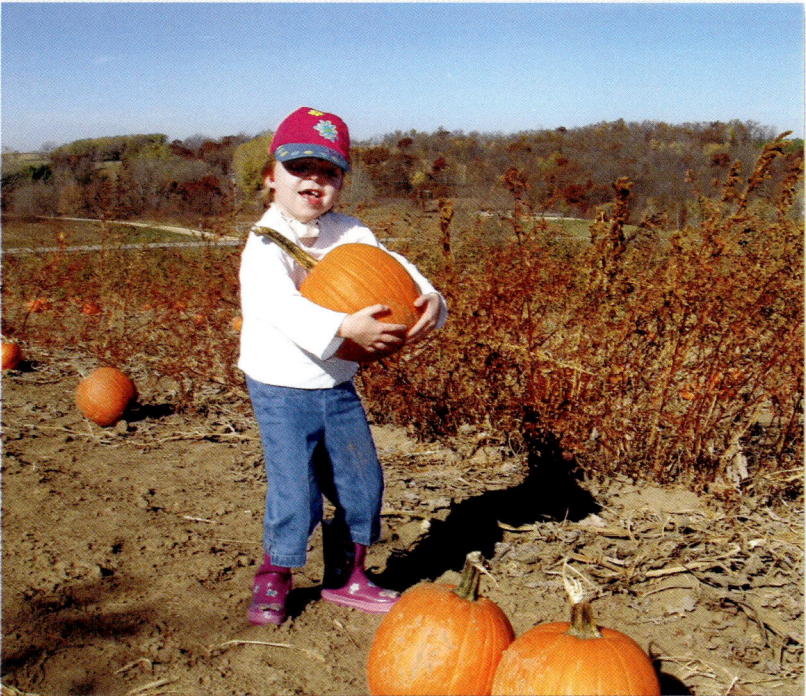

Ellie in a pumpkin patch (2003)

Dear Parent,
When your child was born, you made a very hard choice.

This choice would change the course of your life and challenge you in ways you didn't think it was possible to be challenged.

Yet you pushed on. Within a couple years, you learned how to troubleshoot machines, watch for symptoms, ask the right questions and ignore the wrong ones. You became a "special needs parent."

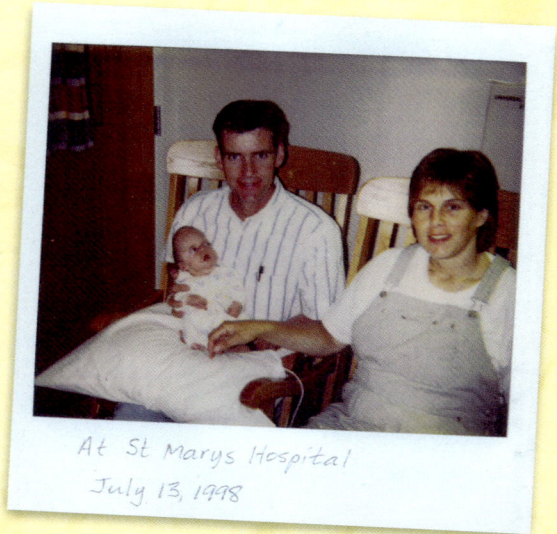

At St Marys Hospital
July 13, 1998

There are days when you see other families doing activities that your family cannot do, and it hurts. It hurts to think about what could-have-should-have-been and it hurts to think of the life you previously lead.

But when you then look at your family, imagining anything different seems almost impossible.

As your child grows, you'll be amazed at their strength, their tenacity, and their ability to push through, no matter what life throws at them—and I hope you know that it all comes from you.

You were the first person in your child's life. You're the person they've turned to for strength and guidance. They've watched you in doctor's offices and hospitals, home and in public.

Whatever face you showed your child is the attitude that will carry them through the rest of their life.

When you made that decision for your child so many years ago, it may have cost you your life—but it gave them theirs.

People *love* to tell me that I'm "brave" or "strong." They say this after I tell them about my craniofacial syndrome and they learn how many surgeries I've had, how long I had braces (nine and a half years), and how much I was questioned and teased in school.

Everybody gives me credit for the way I've persevered, when they should be giving credit to my parents and my sister. My family has had to watch me recover from surgery after surgery, talk to doctors about complications and successes, drive to appointments, sit in waiting rooms, process high levels of information in seconds—all while keeping their emotions hidden. As I've gotten older, I've seen my parents and sister be more transparent about how my medical issues affect them, but I've never seen them break down sobbing (they're usually comforting me as I do that).

I cannot speak for every person with craniofacial syndrome, but I have a feeling that this isn't singular to my experience. I wouldn't be who or where I am today without the lessons my family has taught me.

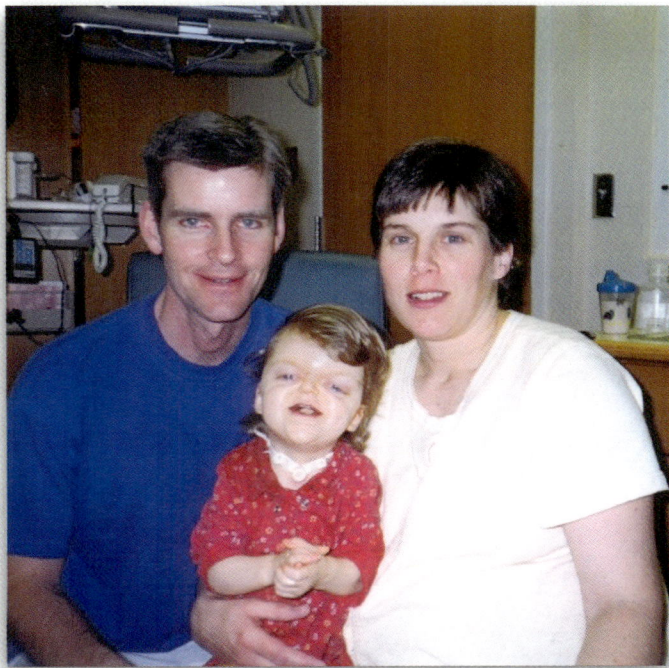

Ellie and her parents in hospital (2000)

IMPORTANCE OF COMMUNITY

A craniofacial syndrome child's quality of life depends more on the community that raises them than on the medical issues that afflict them. If a craniofacial child is raised in a community where they are perceived as "weak" or "different" because of their syndrome, that is all they will ever be. Conversely, if a child is perceived as "strong" and "smart," they'll grow up believing they can conquer the world.

People often like to call children with craniofacial syndromes "brave" or "amazing" for going through all that they have. While those people aren't *wrong*, they're not completely *right* either. It does take a certain amount of strength and stamina to endure surgeries, stares, and everything else that comes with craniofacial syndromes, but without a community to teach a child how to conquer and overcome their struggles, they'll never be able to do so. Craniofacial kids are only as strong as the communities that raise them. Without strong foundations, buildings topple. Without strong communities, craniofacial children fail to thrive.

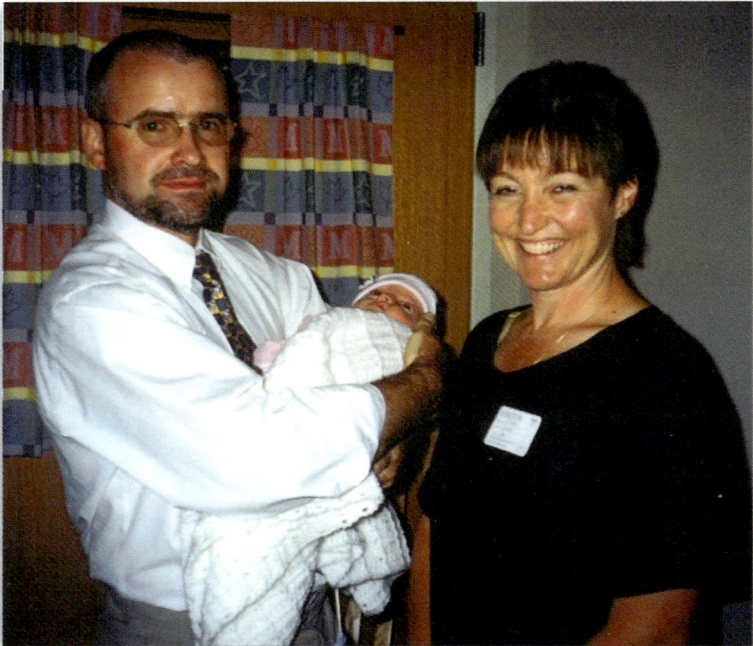

Ellie and her godparents (1998)

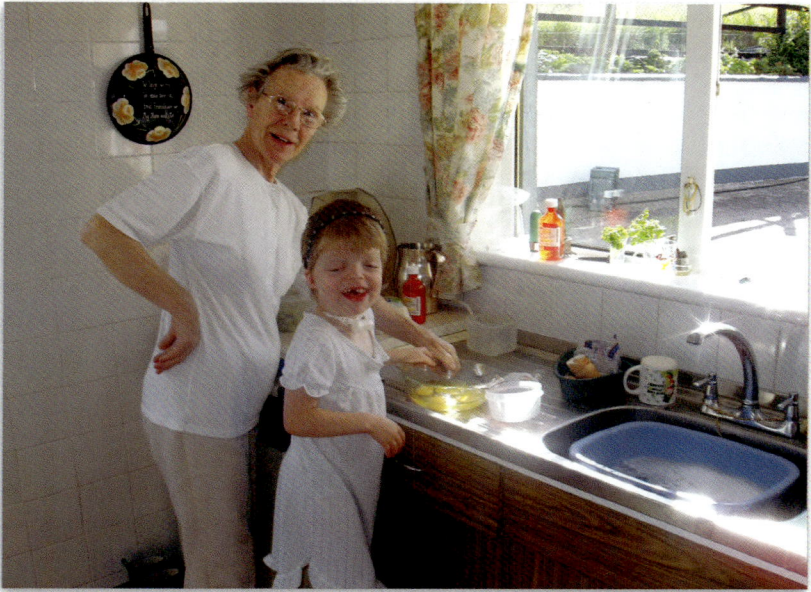

Ellie and her paternal grandmother (2003)

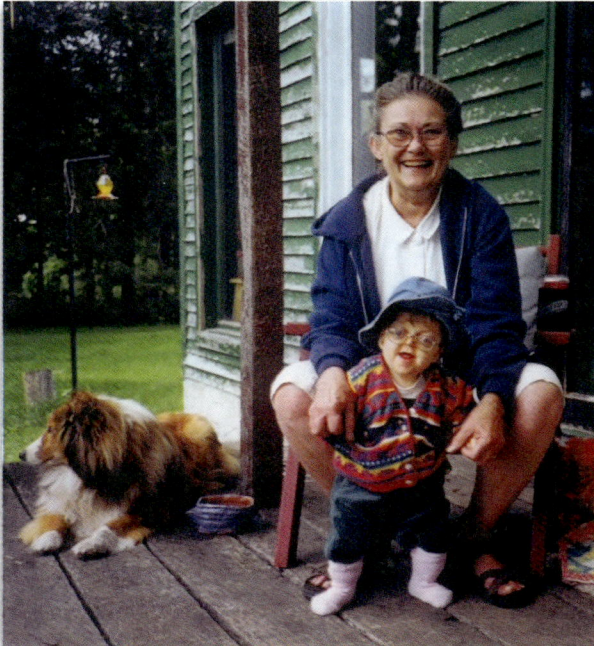

Ellie and her maternal grandmother (1999)

THE WORST THING

Being raised in the Christian faith meant religion every week. Despite being a "Christian atmosphere," the people there were not kind. The girls were cliquey and rude, and the boys pretended to be hotshots. I begged my mom to stop taking me after the first session, yet every Thursday at 6:00 p.m., I found myself being shuttled out the door to a place where I was not welcome or wanted.

One night, after I took my food to a table away from the group, I heard the whispers, "You go talk to her!" "Why not you?" "Okay, I'll go." I could feel my face warming up; I hated when this happened. I kept my head down, but I could feel her walking toward me. She invited me to her table and as I sat with them, we made idle chitchat, and then she scooted closer: "Hey, what's wrong with your face?"

There it was: The Question. Experience had taught me to expect it, but that didn't make me hate it any less. I remember my mom telling me after one of my surgeries that I looked beautiful. Did I? Did I really look beautiful, or just acceptable? If I looked beautiful, why were people being so mean? Aren't I more than my outward appearances?

When we were told to pick a movie to watch for the evening, I rejoiced. It was a moment when I wouldn't have to socialize with these people. The leaders dimmed the lights and hushed the boys being rowdy in the back, and the movie began. The movie was a peaceful time; nobody was talking, and I had found a girl to sit with who—for once—didn't ask The Question. Suddenly, a boy turned around. He had bright ginger hair, blue eyes, and lots of freckles. "What's wrong with your face?" Really? If I didn't answer it the first bazillion times, I'm not going to answer it now. Besides, doesn't the Bible tell us not to judge?

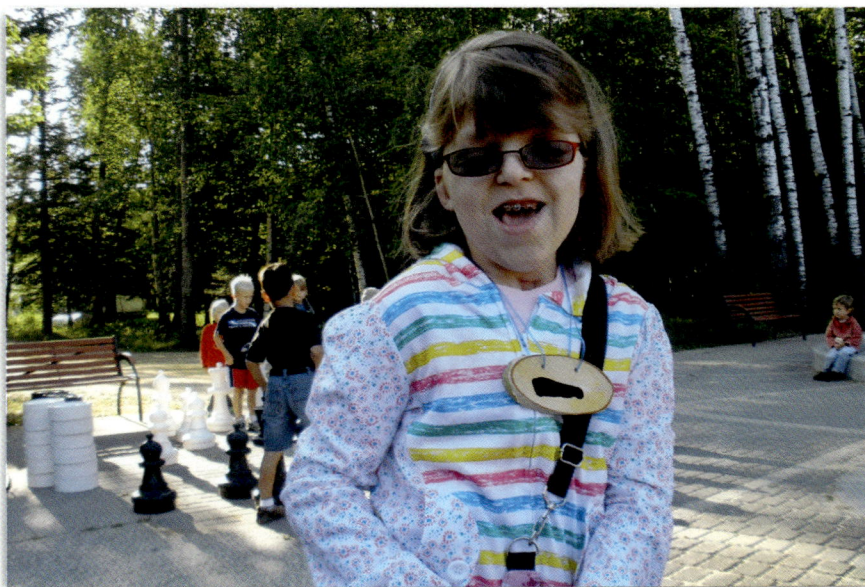
Ellie at summer camp (2008)

Because saying "none of your business" was somehow considered "rude," I had been taught some "polite" responses to The Question: "I was born like this" and "God made me this way." When, for a second time, he asked, "What's wrong with your face?" I responded, "It's the way God made me." It didn't work. For a final time—louder—he asked, "What is wrong with your face?" But before I had a chance to respond, the boy continued, saying, "It is disgusting!"

I couldn't breathe. Conversations that had been happening nearby stopped. All eyes were on us. Even though I felt like I had been kicked in the stomach, I went to tell the leader what he had said.

I remember my mom telling me after one of my surgeries that I looked beautiful. Did I? Did I really look beautiful, or just acceptable? If I looked beautiful, why were people being so mean? Maybe I'm nothing more than what people call me.

Dear Doctor,

I was born with craniofacial syndrome and have had over seventeen surgeries in twenty years. I've seen many doctors in many places; some have been amazing and others have not. One of the worst experiences that I'd like to tell you about was a craniofacial conference in Los Angeles. For hours, different doctors came and went, talked to my parents, yet never acknowledged their patient—me—by name. Instead, I was identified as "she," "her," or "the patient." The best part of the day is when the last doctor came to see me, squatted down, and simply said, "Hi Ellie!" To that one doctor, I was a person worth acknowledging, not just a name on a chart to write off.

Doctor, you have a lot of things to do before the day is done, but that does not excuse you from being rude. You have many patients to see and think about, but that does not give you permission to ignore the ten-year-old in your presence right now. Before you greet your patient, make sure they are the only thing on your mind. Greet them—no matter their age or abilities—with a smile. Address them by name. Regardless of whatever else is on your mind, it is your job to care for them—so make sure you let them know that.

They may not understand your words, but they sure as hell understand your actions.

Sincerely,

Ellie Rose

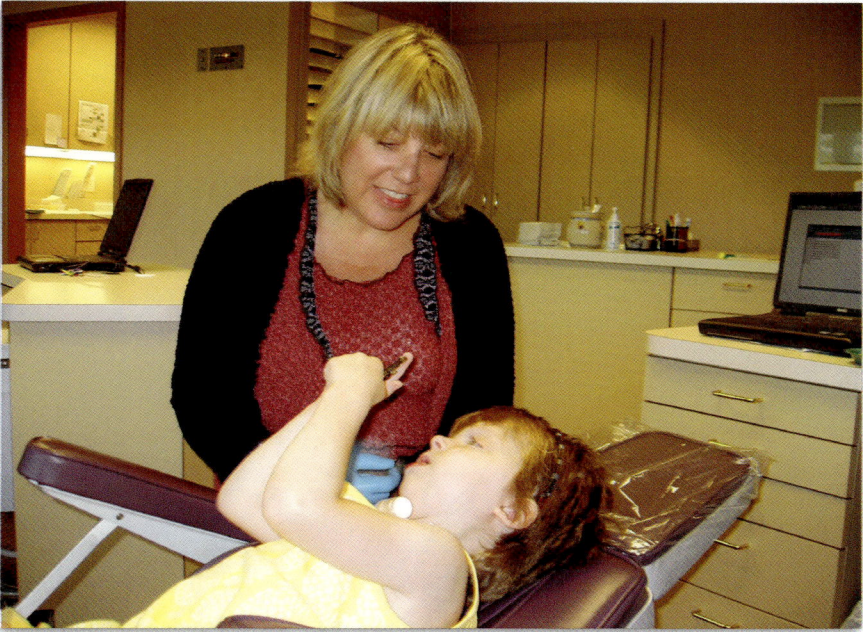
Ellie and one of her pediatric orthodontists (2003)

MY GREATEST ACHIEVEMENT

The first time I called myself pretty, I didn't look at my full-body reflection: I looked myself in the eyes.

Up to this point, I had spent the majority of my life hating the way I looked. I was insecure about every aspect of my face, and if ever I was called "pretty," I thought it was a lie.

In 2009, I had a craniofacial surgery and my face changed dramatically. The doctor told my mom to be careful with me in public because people would stare at me (and they did). This only served as confirmation of something I already knew: I was different and different was bad.

In high school, I moved to a new school where nobody stared and nobody asked questions. At one point, someone gave me a handshake and told me I looked like someone worth getting to know. That comment was earth-shattering. Hearing that phrase flipped a switch in my brain, and while the resentment I had toward my face wasn't eliminated, it was weakened.

In 2016, I had another craniofacial surgery and again my face changed dramatically. At some point, the doctor told my parents, "she's cute." Mom relayed this information to me, and while I didn't believe it, I held onto it.

While recovering from surgery, I started college. Something about the environment I was in changed the way I saw myself. I remember waking up one morning and looking at my face—my bright eyes, my jawline (which was just starting to reappear from the swelling), my smile, and my face as a whole, beautiful feature—and I said, "I'm pretty."

I felt so light. Light and loved with the realization that my face was a beautiful part of me, not a bad one. I carried myself with a new confidence and I viewed the world through a more brightly colored lens than I had before. Nothing was off limits to me—I could do anything I wanted, and my face wasn't going to stop me.

I call this my greatest achievement. Coming to the realization that I am pretty changed my life forever.

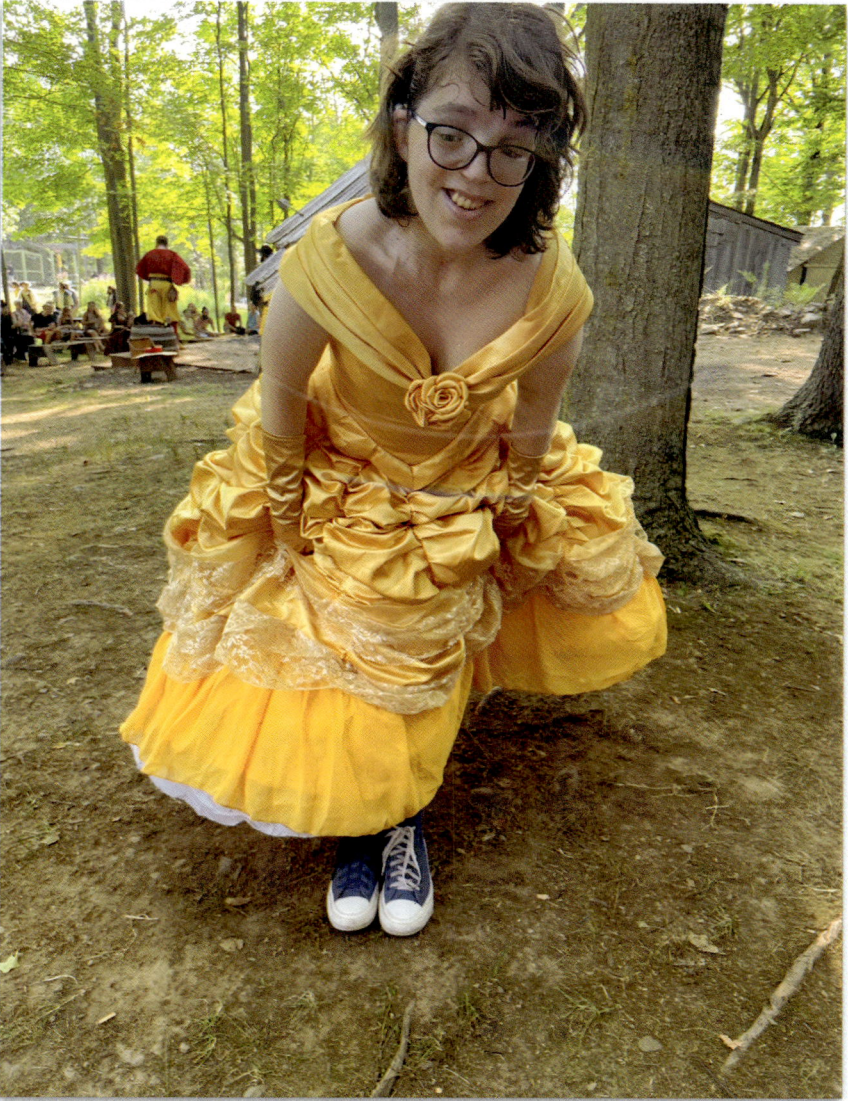
Ellie dressed as Princess Belle for a Renaissance Faire (2021)

Ellie,

Before the time you turn eighteen, you will know that you look different. However, you know now that "different" doesn't mean bad. You'll start talking and writing about what you've been through, sharing the humor in your journey as well as the struggles you've faced. While recovering from surgery, you'll call yourself "pretty" for the first time and you'll feel lighter and brighter than ever before.

By the time you turn twenty-two, you will realize that your precious smile brightens every room you enter. Although you still get stared at, it doesn't measure up to the way your bright blue eyes light up when you're making people laugh or talking about your passions.

By the time you're twenty-five, you will have been kissed and called "cute" and "pretty" (which you never thought would happen). You still feel your insecurities from time to time, but they don't limit you the way they once did.

I couldn't be prouder of who you've become.

You are so beautiful, and I'm so glad you know that. Your smile is contagious, and your confidence can fill a room. You've been through hell and back and made it to the other side—and, my goodness, isn't it magnificent?

You used to distance yourself from the world because you didn't want to get hurt, but now you embrace the world and all it has to offer. When people ask questions, you see it as an opportunity to teach others about conditions they might not know about. You've been vulnerable to life's cruelties and it took a while before you let your guard down. With time, grace, and strength, you've become a force to be reckoned with.

You have done amazing things, Ellie Rose. You're destined to do many more.

Sincerely,

A Friend

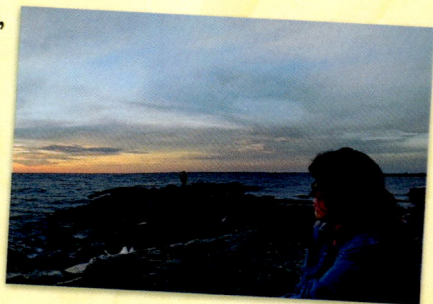

Ellie by Lake Ontario (2022)

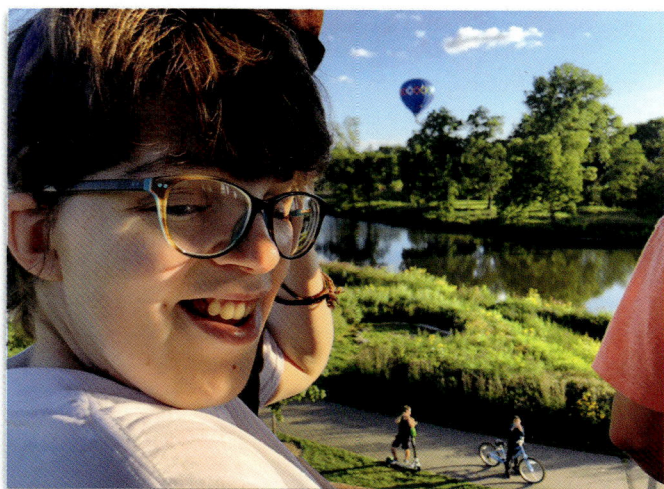
Ellie in a hot air balloon (2021)

EPILOGUE

According to my mom, when I was around seven, I turned to her when we were in a bookstore and said, "I'm gonna write a page-turner one day."

As a kid, I read fictional books about people who never had to be in the hospital. Characters without a hearing aid, or scars. They never knew what it felt like to sit in a hospital waiting room, terrified of the upcoming surgery and cranky because they were fasting and hungry. Characters who seemed to fall in love easily, and who never seemed to care what they looked like. I couldn't be those characters, and I hated it.

I don't remember when I heard the quote, "if there's a book that you want to read, but it hasn't been written yet, then you must write it" (later I learned that it was said by Toni Morrison), but I remember it clicked something in my brain. I had gotten sick of reading about characters who were nothing like me, so I started writing fictional stories about characters with scars, hearing aids, and glasses and who knew what an IV pump sounded like—just like me.

I have been given a gift in that I am a good writer, and I don't intend on letting that gift go to waste. This is my first (mini) memoir, but it certainly will not be my last. There is magic in writing, and being able to share my stories and experiences has connected me with so many people. To see how my stories can change and/or impact people—and how other people change and impact me—is incredible.

Onto the next chapter…

ACKNOWLEDGMENTS

To Dr. Hinda Mandell and RIT Press for giving me the opportunity to accomplish a goal I've had since I was a wee girl—thank you so much.

Mom, Dad, and Orla—Thank you for not letting me be defined by my face and showing me that I am capable of conquering the world. These stories would not be possible without the love, laughs, and support I have received from you.

Abby Christena, Andrew Bernard, Benjamin Louis, Matthew Joseph, and Vera Eris—With grace, love, and tomfoolery, you've helped me become the woman I am today: a published author!

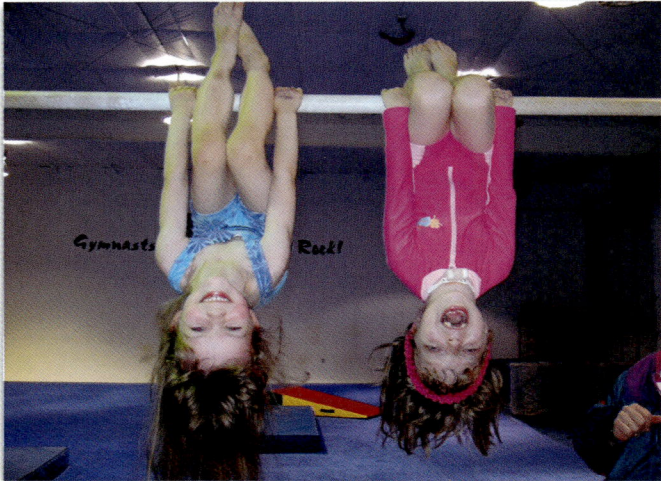

Ellie and her younger sister Orla at gymnastics (2004)

ABOUT THE AUTHOR

Ellie Rose McCullagh was born with a craniofacial syndrome that has required over twenty surgeries on her face, skull, brain, and airway. She is in her last year of studies at RIT and is hoping to graduate in May 2025. Using what she has learned in the School of Individualized Study (SOIS), McCullagh is hoping to pursue social science research and somehow integrate her experiences in the medical field into her long-term goals—whatever they may be. In addition to being a student, McCullagh is also a musician, writer, artist, and coffee lover.